Beyond The Wilderness

P.M.HILL

chipmunkapublishing
The mental health publisher

All rights reserved, no part of this publication may be reproduced by any means, electronic, mechanical photocopying, documentary, film or in any other format without prior written permission of the publisher.

Published by
Chipmunkapublishing
United Kingdom

http://www.chipmunkapublishing.com

Copyright © 2018 P.M.HILL

ISBN   978-1-78382-397-0

LOVE YOU **MUM**

I love you mum
Though you're not around anymore
You knew the score
And a strictness
I could not ignore
But the grounding second to none.
I forgive you mum.

YOU DIDN'T LIKE YOUR MOTHER DID YOU?

You didn't like your mother
A dying father said.
The son paused
And then he replied

It wasn't so much my lack of love
Or the lack of love from her

It wasn't the lack of clothes,
toys, birthdays, holidays,
and Christmas cheer.

It was more… it was more about…

There wasn't a hoop I could jump through
A degree I could earn,
A change I could make,
A job I could do.

That would help her talk to me in a way
That said I love you

Always that hectoring tone
That expressed emotion,
That disapproving look

Always the fear of her raised vice
That cold expression
That look of disgust
Always feeling I was or about to be
In trouble.

Dressed for bed time at four pm.

Mess is not good.

Clothes must always be clean,
The house always be tidy.

But.

Can children play in tidy clean houses,

Without throwing stones,

Without feeling dead inside.

P.M.Hill

YOU'RE NOT TOO TO BE HIT BOY

You're not to big to be hit boy

I've got a stick outside,
One more word from you boy,

And it's ten whacks on the backside.

Seen and not heard
That's what children should be,
Unseen and heard
Would bring anarchy.

Your eyes are bigger than
Your belly
How dare you not like my jam,

Eat or else it's no jelly
And another sulk
And it's nothing on the telly.

You can't have the faggot gravy
And butter on your spuds,

Like custard and cream on your pudding,
It simply isn't done,

If you don't eat your dinner,
There'll be no pudding

And

Ignore the ring of the ice cream van
It doesn't toll for you,

Another noise out of place and it's the end for me and you.

Great family traditions.

Mother and father met in All Saints
All those years ago.

Named us after
Biblical characters,

Matthew,Mark, and John and Peter
And Anita.!!??

An aunt called Jess,
Didn't have the such lineage

But

Joined the tradition too.

Her head was slapped against
A drainpipe,

So she became
Obsessive Compulsive too.

Trendsetter in every way our great grandma was,

To be a single parent in 1920s
Birmingham,

She must have felt a bit of a fool

It certainly wasn't cool

Kids by four fathers

Dare I say it ,
Dare I say it.

You could be…..

Put away in
All Saints for such so called misdemeanors.

THE WOMAN AT THE JOB CENTRE SAID I HAS SCHIZOPHRENIA.

The woman at the job centre said I had schizophrenia,

'That's what they think'
My mother said.

You're not the same though
You're not the same.

Since you arrived back in Birmingham

I think they bought back someone else

You're not the same person
We took to Leicester.

I think in fact you're an imposter,

You're slow, you're sleepy,

You just don't have the get up and go..

In fact there's not much you now know

I say, 'Get a grip, young man, and in the great scheme
Of things.'

'Pull yourself together,

'I think it written in your genes.

I'M NOT DYING AM I?

'I'm not dying am I.'

A mother said to dad.

Tubes and monitors everywhere

To avoid the scare.

'Course not' he said.

He did want her to know he did care.

Looking up she saw the bearded one,

Crying at the foot of the bed.

She drifted out of consciousness

Once more

A child's voice

Then the call , the call of Mum.

'I love you. I love you'

The dying woman said.

Reaching out to those left behind.

Leaving the world a better, better place.

Remorse in kind.

IRONING BOARD JUSTICE.

The prosecutor, judge and jury

The fate of the boys to be decided

'You're selfish'

'All you think about is number one'

The ironing board mother said.

Judge Jess stood, iron in hand,

Like mothers do across the land?

' The boys sat waiting'

For hours

For the weekly verdict on their
Misdemeanours.

And so she went on and.

And on and on.

Count by count the charges were read.

And not content till ' till' the boys'

Took heed and pleaded guilty to every naughty deed.

Then the silence as Judge Jess
Took account of the evidence,

She then deferred the sentence,

She sought instead to build them back up
At the double,

Recognising no one infallible,

She said that was laughable

And the Judge Jess and 'the boys then briefly parted

She laughed when one of them farted.

And so it was.

And so it was.

Lashings of butter and malt loaf and tea.

'The boys' and mother laughed in glee.

NOT LIKE HIS MOTHER!!

'Not like his mother' a foster mum said

Now he was ill in the head.

She remembered that time ... that time

When visiting his mother

In that padded cell.

She didn't want a repeat of that to her son.

They said he didn't even know

His name.

To be a strong mother had been her aim.

But now the tears she shed.

She wished she could hug that head.

P.M.Hill

UNCLE PHILIPS BETTER MUMMY?

'Uncle Philips better mummy.

A young girl said.

For thirty years

He had been ill in the head.

That foggy look.
That vacant stare.

Now uncle Philip would take time to care.

BIG SISTER

You weren't so big once big sister.

You looked or should I say I looked down on you.

Now I call on your wisdom

Daily too often as I do.

A friend in need is a pest and add to that
A soulmate too.

Your knowledge of child development

Is somewhat intricate

That's the last time toys with knobs on.

 Or relate to a six year old in abstract terms
That really isn't on.

Your patience is endless, your diplomacy discrete,
nothing can seem to shift you off those

Novelty slippered feet

Your judgement is sound

Your knowledge abounds,

The discerning nature is clear.

I-have nothing to fear

Big sister.

P.M.Hill

YOU'LL BE A MAN MY SON.

(A hypothetical final from father to son)

I told you once you were my son
I told you once that you were precious
I told you I would never disown you
Or betray you
Whatever you did
Or said or thought
And so it is my son
As I approach the end
I was never discouraged

When you balled at your mum
Mistreated your brother
Or sulked in endless fashion
Such were the growing pains
Me myself made a man by the army
You yourself graduated to the same height
You were my son
Even when pupils bullied
And insulted you
When you you ran like a coward
When you fell in love
With the idea of falling in love and had a breakdown
You were still my son

I was never disappointed
During that thirty year fog
That chemical straight jacket
I lived to see you
Break those shackles free
To find the real you
And I embraced that
To see the very you shine through

But don't implode over my demise
You'll still be my son when I am gone
Still I will guide you. Nurture you, Protect you.
Love not because of what you do, think or say
I love because you are mine.

Beyond The Wilderness

There was a time when
Your humanity was under construction
A rite of passage it may have been
But since that rebirth
You became a friend and Dwelt within me
Just as I did in you

And what's more. You are a man my son.

Philip Hill

Loving son.

DADS MEMORY TEST.

Father ruler

Boy in hand

Players on wall

Brummie land

'At the back'

'Combes, Robson, Ross, Aitken and Nicholl,

The boy recited

He got them all right,

So they were both delighted.

At the front,

The ruler went,

'Graydon, Rioch, and Little

And that man in tracksuit dad'

'Manager son'

He retorted

'Crowe' he got the first name distorted.

In the middle the ruler jabbed,

',Not a clue, Son.'

The boy thoughts pausing a while,

His thoughts frozen,

The midfield not chosen,
'Anderson!! Hamilton!! And Godfrey, Son.

Remember the names and don't be be scared and

Next time be better prepared.

FATHER IN CYBERSPACE.

Dad,

You don't talk to me now,
About the Villa, The Cottage, or the garden,

You don't tell me to cut my cloth to my
Budget,

To stop being harsh to my kid
brother.

To chide me with caution about my dodgier fb, blogs.

But before you died.

I told you how much you would be missed.

I told you of how proud I was …

To be…. To be., 'King of Dads'

And so it is dad, my friend, my advocate, my confidante.

Nothing was left unsaid
No unexpressed doubts,

No more grounding in reality.

No more needing to, 'get a grip'.

You died a grandad to some, a dad to us, and an
Estranged brother and somehow

I was ready….. ready….

To be that responsible brother, uncle, and friend,
To those left behind.

I miss your affirmation most,
Your fab blogs to say you were proud.

I told you I loved you.

'And I love you too, unconditionally, son.'

Came the fb reply,

I dared to say the unsayable
When I dared to ask if I had been a 'let down'

'A let down! A let down.'

'No, no son, you just had a tragic life'.

A 101 SHEEP.

All the sheep
In a pen,

Stood

Waited

Gate open.

Master and dog

In a rush

All two

Absent,

Restless

Searching

A wanderer

By a cliff edge?

Solitary

Lonely

Breathing

Beyond The Wilderness

Wanderer

Take my hand

You know I'll be there

I'll cross the see for you

And the ends of the earth

Take, take my hand

And I'll lead you

Your were lost but are now found

Trapped, but now

Beyond hope?

But now rescued

Don't look at me

Wanderer

I am more than you can

Bear, just…..just.

Be still and know that

I am there for you.

Don't think

Just be still

Look at your feet

And walk

Only… only
When you see the step ahead

Wait.. wait.

Be still

I will show you the way

I left a hundred sheep waiting

Still

For you

Better unattended

Than a single lost soul

Better to knock, ask and search

And lose yourself for a moment in life

Than never find yourself.

www.ingramcontent.com/pod-product-compliance
Ingram Content Group UK Ltd.
Pitfield, Milton Keynes, MK11 3LW, UK
UKHW041413180426
11947UKWH00007B/117